What is this book about

This book is a cook book filled with favourite party foods and refreshments. It will be a helpful hand for you to organise your party foods in no time. It offers you the most popular Asian cuisines designed with healthy ingredients such as coconut oil, Coconut milk, coconut flakes, and spices authentic to Asian flavours.

Why I wrote this book

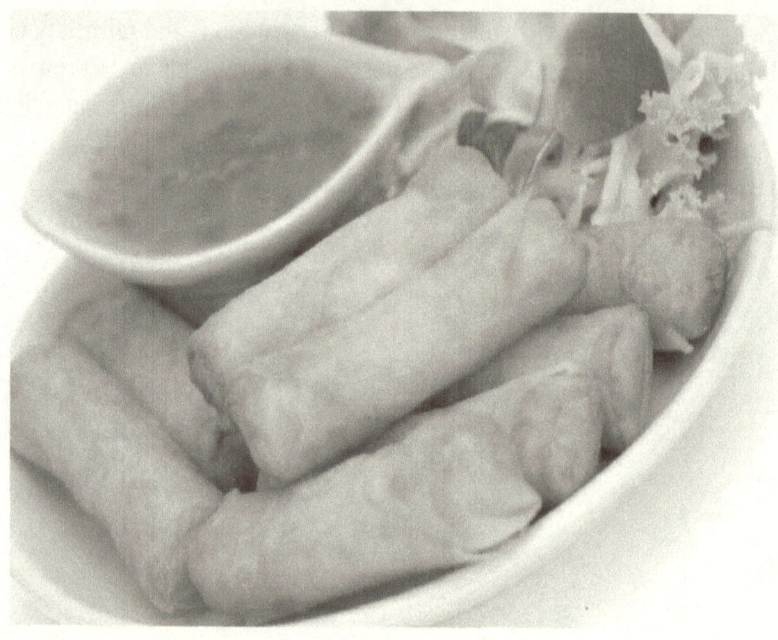

I wrote this book because I wanted to share my knowledge about Asian cooking to people who are willing to learn about the art of these mouth-watering recipes .Nowadays people are migrating to different countries and the values, cultures, especially food that are authentic to Asians are diminishing. Most people who live in overseas are craving to try these recipes but do not know the exact recipes , measurements and method to try them out .. I realized the importance of cherishing these lovely traditional cooking for our future generations. I wanted to share my experience and knowledge .This inspired me to write this book.

I know learning the correct method of how to cook these yummy foods is not easy without knowing the right method, ingredients, and quantities.

I went through the same tough time by myself until I knew what is right for my taste buds. The things I learnt and saw 20 years ago have changed with the new technologies and new cultural changes. Hence I wanted to share my knowledge about these amazing Asian cooking to people who are willing to learn about the art of these mouth-watering recipes.

Why you should read this book

The **goal** of "Coconut Oil Recipes" is to **share my secrets about Asian cuisines to wider audience.** The recipes I have carefully selected will enlighten and entertain both the Western and Asians taste buds. These recipes offer healthy ingredients such as coconut oil, coconut milk, coconut flakes, and spices to add authentic Asian flavours and great for parties, as a snack or for any occasion.

Now a day these recipes are very popular not only among Asians but also European and North American countries. Hence this book will appeal **both Asian and Western Taste buds**. Also these days' people are more interested in healthy cooking. These recipes are mostly made out of Coconut oil, Coconut flakes, Coconut Milk and spices. According to research coconut is named as a super food. This designation is due to its unique combination of fatty acids that have profound positive effects on health.

This book will appeal to people who like **healthy cooking** since it is filled with different recipes with coconut oil, coconut milk, coconut flakes, and spices authentic to Asian flavours, hence most of the food lovers who like to experiment different foods will attract this book.

Table of Contents

Patties (Deep fried pastries)
Chinees Rolls
Egg Rolls
Fish Buns (Malu Paan)
Rainbow Sandwich
Aloo Bonda
Cutlets
Seeni Sambal Buns (Spicy stir-fried Onion buns)
Prawns wade –Isso Wade
Masala Wade
Ulundu Wade
Coconut Chutney
Vegetable or Fish Roti (Gothamber Roti)
Egg Roti / Vegetarian Roti
Egg Sandwiches
Chicken Sandwiches
Sweets
    Coconut Toffee/ Coconut Rocks
    Milk Toffees / Caramel Fudge
    Potato Toffees/ Potato Fudge
    Marshmallows
    Meringues/Kisses
    MURRUKKU
    Doughnuts

Patties (Deep fried pastries)

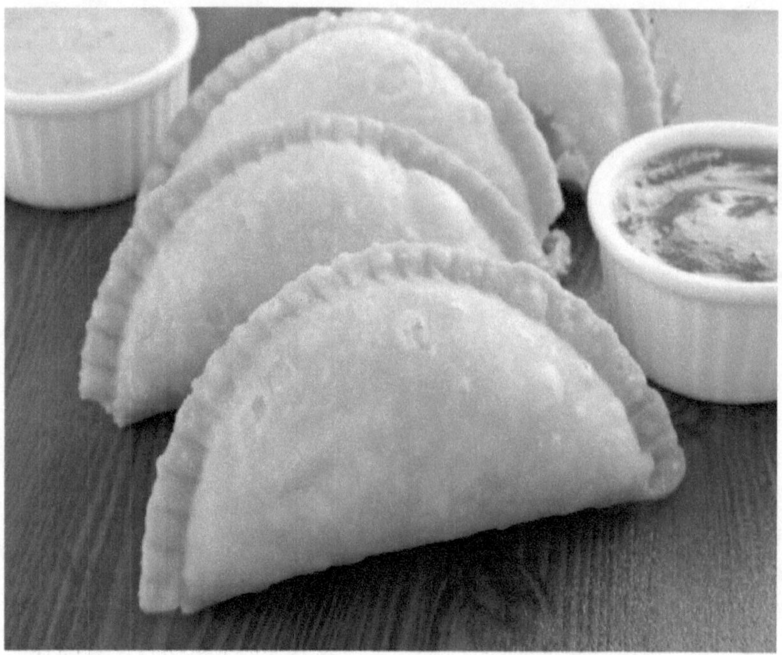

(30-35 Patti's)

Ingredients for dough:

- 250 g plain flour (2 Cups)
- 60 ml water
- 115g Chilled Butter
- ½ Bottle Coconut oil for frying
- You can use the same cutlet filling or use the following filling

Dough -Method

Mix the chilled butter with flour and beat it with an electric mixer for 30 seconds .Then add the 60ml chilled water little by little and kneed for 10 minutes until the pastry becomes a non-stick smooth dough. Leave the dough in the fridge for 15 minutes.

(Meanwhile you can make the filling)

After 15 minutes roll the dough on a flour dusted board. Cut the dough in to half and roll it through a rolling pin into a thin pastry. About 1/8 inch thickness. Use a round cutter or a glass and cut round circles. Put a spoonful of the filling into the middle, fold it in to half .Wet the edges with water and seal the edges by pressing with a fork leaving the fork marks nicely. Deep fry patties in the coconut oil until golden brown and serve hot.

Filling

- 425g potatoes
- 1 big onion finely chopped
- 1 can of Salmon or Jack mackerel-425g (or Leaks and carrots for vegetarian filling)
- 3 green chillies finely chopped
- 6-8 curry leaves
- 1/2 lime
- 2 Tsp pepper to taste
- ½ Tsp Chilli powder
- ½ tsp Curry Powder
- Salt to taste

(If you don't like chilli and curry powder you can omit that and use only pepper powder)

Make filling: (for vegetarian recipe)

Mashes the potatoes leave aside .Finely chop the leeks and carrots set aside. Stir fry the onions in oil in a pan for about 4-5mins under low heat. Add the vegetables and stir fry for a few more minutes. Add the curry powder and chilli powder. Fry for a minute. Add the potatoes. Add salt and pepper to taste. Set aside.

Make filling: (for fish recipe)

Flake the salmon. Mash the potatoes leave aside .Stir fry the onions in oil in a pan for about 4-5mins under low heat. Add the fish and stir fry for a few

more minutes. Add the curry powder and chilli powder. Fry of a minute. Add
the potatoes. Add salt and pepper to taste. Set aside.

Chinees Rolls

Delicious snack for tea times or for parties

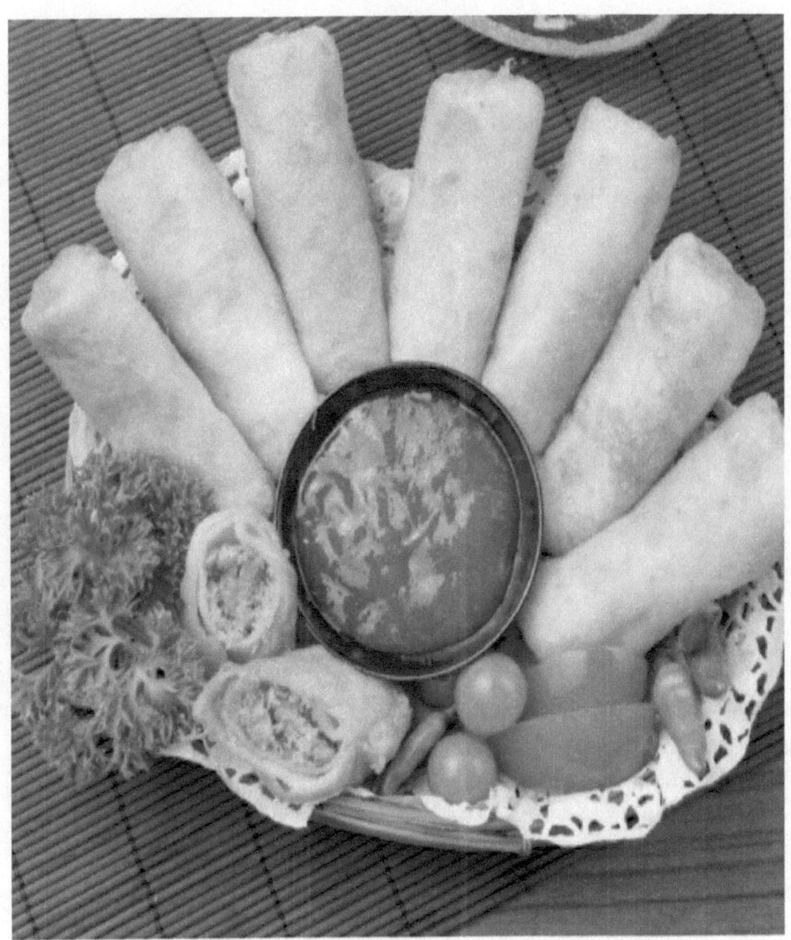

Ingredients

- 225g Flour (2 Cups)
- 2 Cups Water
- 2 Eggs
- 1 Tsp salt

- ½ Bottle of coconut oil for frying
- 2 eggs for the egg wash
- Bread Crumbs for the coating

Filling

- 1 can of Salmon or Jack mackerel-425g (or Leaks and carrots for vegetarian filling) +Boiled eggs if you are making egg rolls
- 400g potatoes
- 1 big onion finely chopped
- 3 green chillies finely chopped
- 4-5 curry leaves chopped
- 1/2 lime
- 2 Tsp Pepper Powder
- 1 Tsp Crushed Chilli powder
- Salt to taste

(If you don't like chilli and curry powder you can omit that and use only pepper powder)

Method

Batter

Mix flour, water, egg, salt together and make a runny and smooth batter. Put 1 tsp coconut oil in a frying pan and when the oil is hot add 1 large spoonful of the mixture into the pan and turn into circular motion and make thin pan cakes and set aside.

Make the filling as for cutlets or patties and set aside. If you are making egg rolls boil the eggs and set aside.

Put the above filling in the middle fold from both edges and then roll it until a fine roll is formed. If you like egg rolls leave a half an egg in the middle with the fish or vegetable filling. Wet the edges with little bit of egg whites and seal it. Dip in a beaten egg and press on bread crumbs and deep fry in coconut oil till golden brown and serve hot.

Egg Rolls

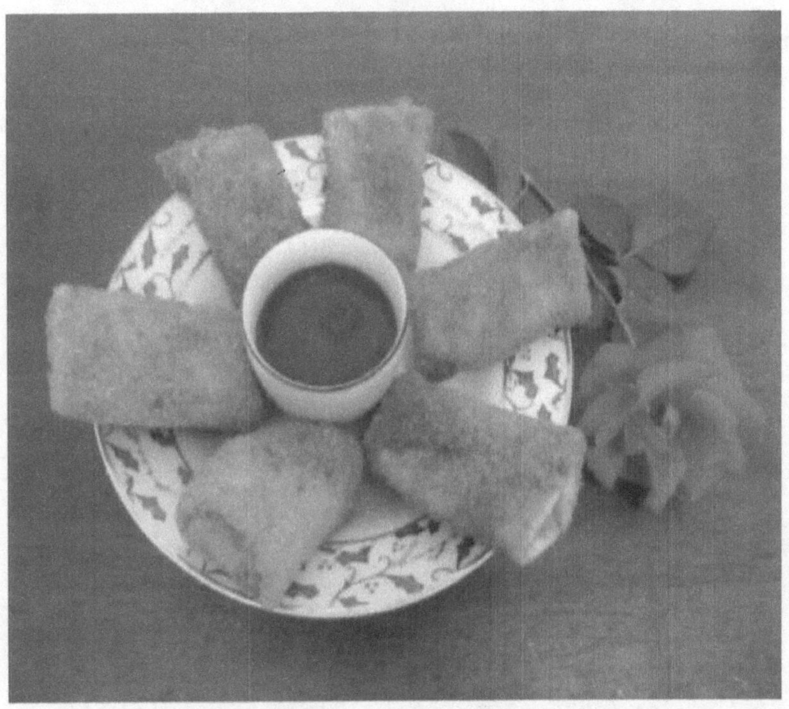

Please follow the same recipe for Chinees rolls. Except add a half of a boiled egg with the fish filling when making the rolls.

Fish Buns (Malu Paan)

Nothing like Sri Lankan Malu Pan as a snack or for parties.

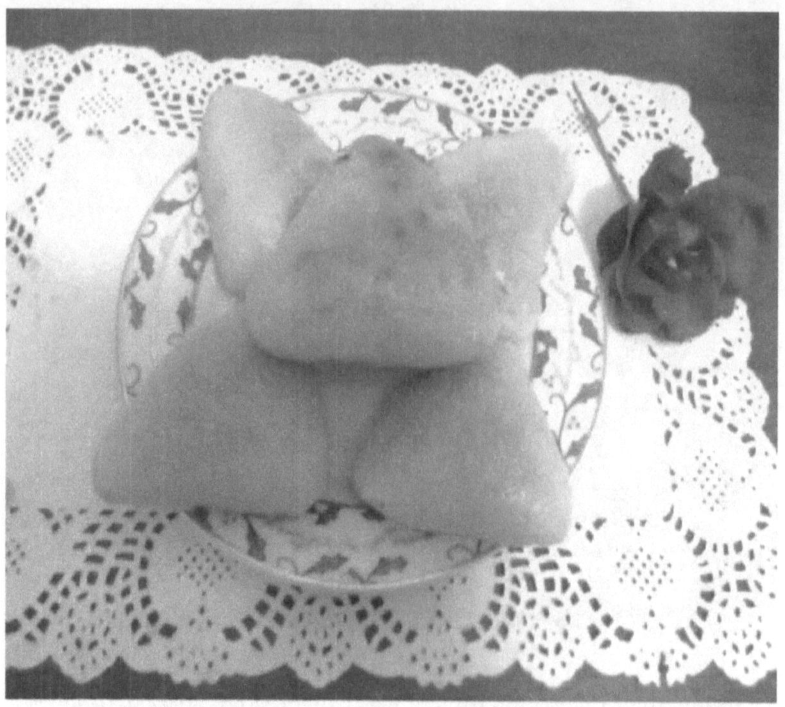

Ingredients

- Dough
- 500 g Flour (plain)
- 1-1/2 tea spoon salt
- 1-1/2 tea spoons sugar
- 1 Satchel of yeast – 7g dry yeast
- 1 1/2 cup moderate warm water

Topping / glazing

- 1 egg

- 1 tea spoon sugar

Filling

- 1 can of Salmon, mackerel or boiled boneless fish -425g
- 500g potatoes
- 1 big onion finely chopped
- 3 green chillies finely chopped
- 2 Tsp pepper powder
- 4-5 curry leaves
- 1/2 lime
- Salt to taste
- 2tbs Coconut oil for frying

(If you like the filling spicy you can add 1tsp pepper, 1-2 tsp chilli powder and 1 tsp curry powder)

Method

Add yeast with 1-1/2 tea spoon of sugar to a cup mix well and add ½ cup Luke warm water and set aside to ferment for 5 minutes .If the yeast is active there will be bubbles forming up.

Meanwhile add flour and salt to a dry mixing bowl and start mixing using an electric mixer .Add the remaining Luke warm water gradually while mixing. When the bubbles start forming adds the yeast mixture also to the dough and mix well. Mix well under low speed for 10 minutes. Non-sticky dough will form after 10 minutes. Sprinkle some flour in another bowl and transfer the dough to that bowl. Sprinkle some flour to the top of the dough as well. Cover the dough with a wet cloth /cling wrap and leave it to rise for 30 minutes.

(Now it's time to make the filling as you like)

After 30 -40 mints dough becomes doubled the size. Transfer the dough to a floured board and knead it another 10 minutes using your hands.

After 10 minutes kneading divide the dough into small balls. You can make about 11 balls.

Spread each ball on a flat board sprinkled with flour and roll the dough and make thin rounds. Place one large spoonful of the prepared filling in the middle and shape the filling into a triangle shape .Fold the three edges like an envelope to cover the 3 areas to make a triangle .Shape it into a triangle shape and leave it in a baking tray for another 10 minutes to rise. Prepare all the bread dough balls like this.

Now for topping/glazing

Mix an egg with 1tsp sugar. Brush the egg wash on top of each bun.

Bake the buns for 20 to 30 mints in 160 degree of Celsius in a pre- heated oven. Bake until the tops become golden brown.

You can make average size of 11 buns.

Filling

Drain the water and smash the fish into small pieces. Boil skin and Mash the potatoes.

Heat 2 tbsp. of Coconut oil in a pan under medium heat. and add the onions, green chillies and curry leaves and fry till the onions are golden brown.

Now add the mashed fish and temper for about 3-5 minutes.

Then add the mashed potatoes and season with salt and pepper. (If you like add chilli powder and curry powder to you taste) and mix well. Remove from heat and add the lime juice to the mixture and mix well.

Rainbow Sandwich

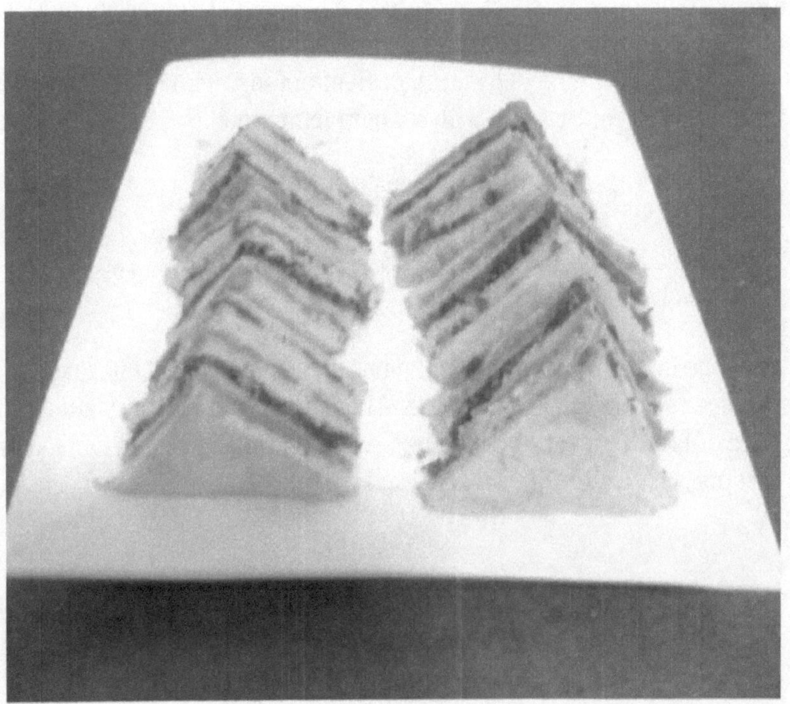

Ingredients

- 2 Carrots Boiled and mashed
- 1 Beetroot Boiled and mashed /Canned beetroot mashed
- 2 Boiled Eggs
- Iceberg Lettuce chopped lengthwise
- Salt and Pepper
- Mustard Cream
- 4 Tsp Coconut Oil
- Lemon Juice
- 1 Sliced loaf of bread

Method

Mix 1 tsp Coconut Oil, Pepper, Salt, ½tsp Mustard and lemon juice to each of Carrot, Beetroot and smashed eggs separately and mix well.

Spread Coconut Oil on 3 slices of bread. You can add 2 thin layers of each of this mixture on the bread and make colourful different sandwiches.Ex: Carrot and eggs or Beetroot mix with carrot, or Beetroot mix with carrot, Beetroot mix with egg mix, or Beetroot with ice burg lettuce etc.

Or you can add 3 layers of the mix in 4 slices of bread.

Ex: You can add Beetroot, carrot, Iceberg lettuce or Beetroot, carrot and egg mix. You can be creative.

Ex: Add one layer of mashed carrot on one slice of bread and one layer of mashed beetroot on one slice of bread. And one layer of ice burg lettuce on one slice of bread. Place them on top of each other. Place buttered bread on top of it press hard and cut the edges. and cut into triangles. Or you can add carrot

Aloo Bonda

This is a great tea time snack.

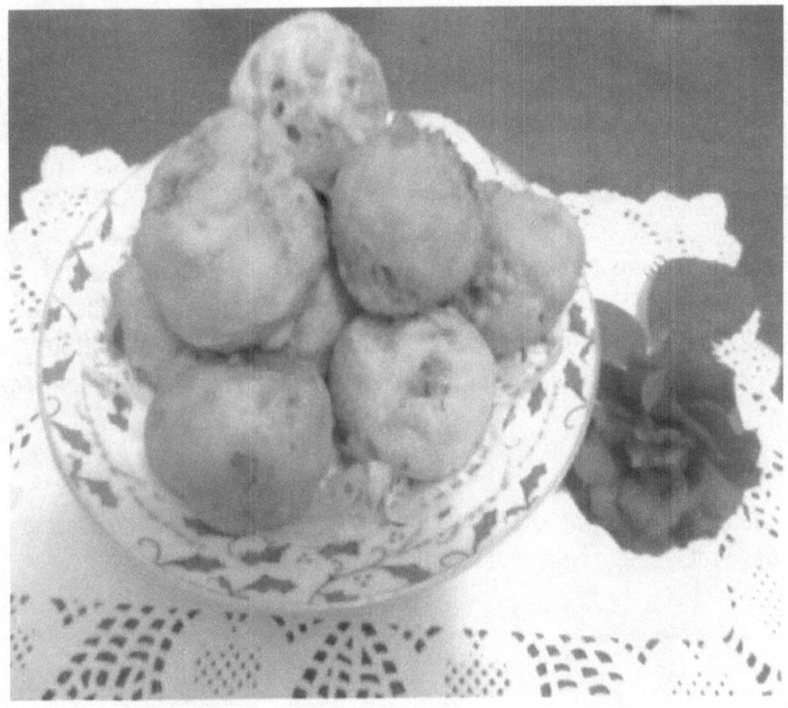

Ingredients

- 500g Potato's Boiled and slightly mashed with small pieces left
- 1 Onion Chopped
- 1 Tsp Mustard Seeds
- 2-3 Green chillies chopped
- 1 Tsp Pepper
- 1 Tsp Turmeric powder
- 1 tsp chopped Coriander and curry leaves
- ½ tsp chopped ginger
- ½ tsp cumin powder
- ½ tsp chili powder

- ½ lemon juice
- Batter
- 1 Cup Chick Pea flour
- ½ cup rice flour
- ½ tsp chilli powder
- ½ tsp baking powder
- ½ bottle coconut oil for frying

Method

Heat 2 Tbsp. oil in a pan and fry add mustard seeds, When mustard seed burst add Onions , Green chillies, chopped coriander, ginger, cumin seeds, salt and turmeric until onion turn into golden colour. Then add the potatoes and cook for 3-4 minutes. Finally add lemon juice. Leave it aside to cool. Once you make the batter as bellow make large handful of balls, dip in plain flour and then in the batter and deep fry until golden brown in colour. Drain and serve.

Batter

Mix the Chick Pea flour, rice flour, turmeric powder, salt and the baking powder .Add enough cold water until it makes a thick batter.

Cutlets

These are delicious as a snack with evening tea or as a side dish for lunch or dinner or any occasion.

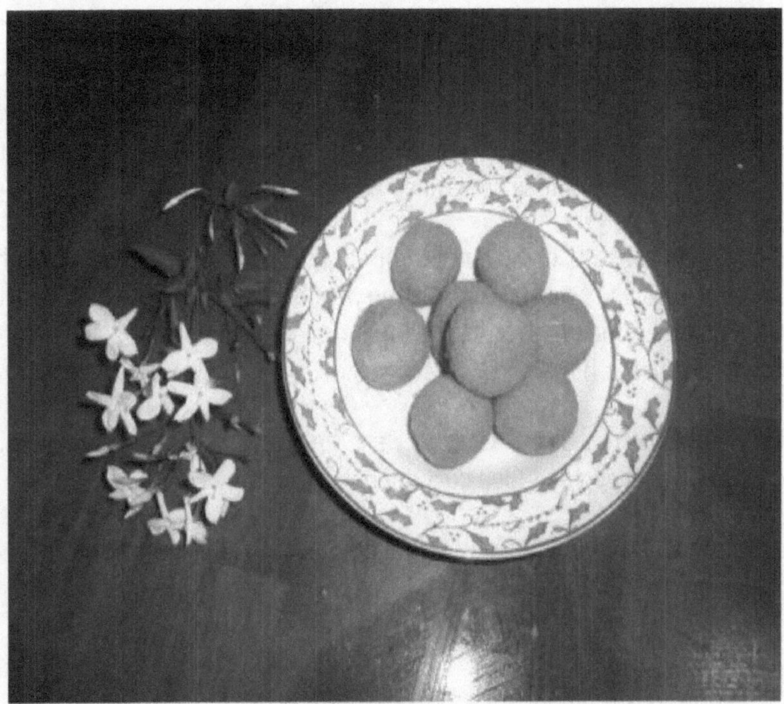

Serves 8-10 people

Ingredients:

- 1 can of Salmon or Jack mackerel-425g or any boneless fish boiled
- 400g potatoes
- 1 big onion finely chopped
- 3 green chillies finely chopped
- 2 Tbsp. Coconut oil
- 1/2 bottle coconut oil for frying
- 4-5 curry leaves

- 1/2 lime
- 1 egg
- 1/4 lb bread crumbs
- Salt and pepper to taste

Method:

Boil skin and Mash the potatoes. Drain the water and smash the fish into small pieces.

Heat 2 tbsp. of oil/ butter in a pan and add the onions, green chillies and curry leaves and fry till the onions are golden brown.

Now add the mashed fish and temper for about 3-5 minutes and then add the mashed potatoes and season with salt and pepper and mix well. Remove from heat and add the lime juice to the mixture and mix well. Once cooled make small balls from the fish mixture. Leave aside.

Leave the bread crumbs in a flat dish. Beat the egg in a bowl. Now soak the balls in the beaten egg and then coat the balls with bread crumbs.

Heat the remaining oil in a frying pan and when the oil is hot add the coated fish balls and fry till golden brown. Makes about 30-40 cutlets. Serve hot.

Seeni Sambal Buns (Spicy stir-fried Onion buns)

Favourite tea time snack as well as party food.

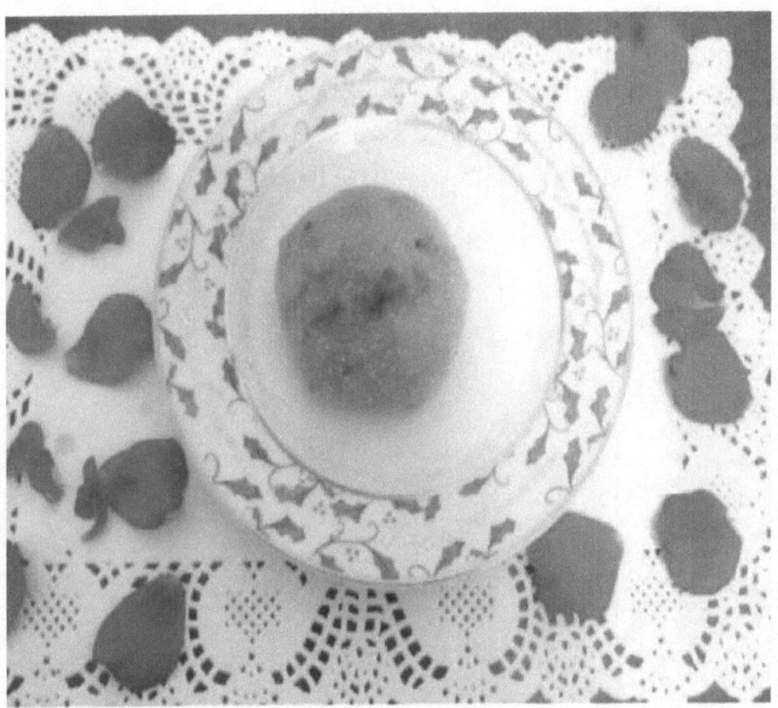

Ingredients

- 500g Flour
- 1 satchels Yeast (7g)
- ¼ Cup Luke warm water
- 1 Tsp salt
- 1 Egg
- 2 Tbsp. Sugar
- ½ Cup Milk
- 2-3 Tbsp. Coconut Oil

Method

Mix the yeast with 2 tbsp. sugar and Luke warm water and set aside to rise. Mix the flour, salt and eggs in a mixing ball and start beating. Once the yeast is risen add this to the flour mix. While beating gradually add milk and 3 tbsp. oil to form into a smooth dough. Beat for 15 minutes. Leave the dough to rise in a warm place for 30 to 40 minutes. Once the dough has risen put it on to a floured board and knead it for 2-3 minutes. Then portion it in to equal sizes. Roll each one of them into a thin circles. Place Seeni Sambal filling in the middle and cover the corners and edges together and roll it into circles. You can also make them as rectangle shapes .leave it to rise for 1 hour. After 1 hour brush the tops with egg wash and put it in the oven 160 for 30 minutes.

Prawns wade –Isso Wade

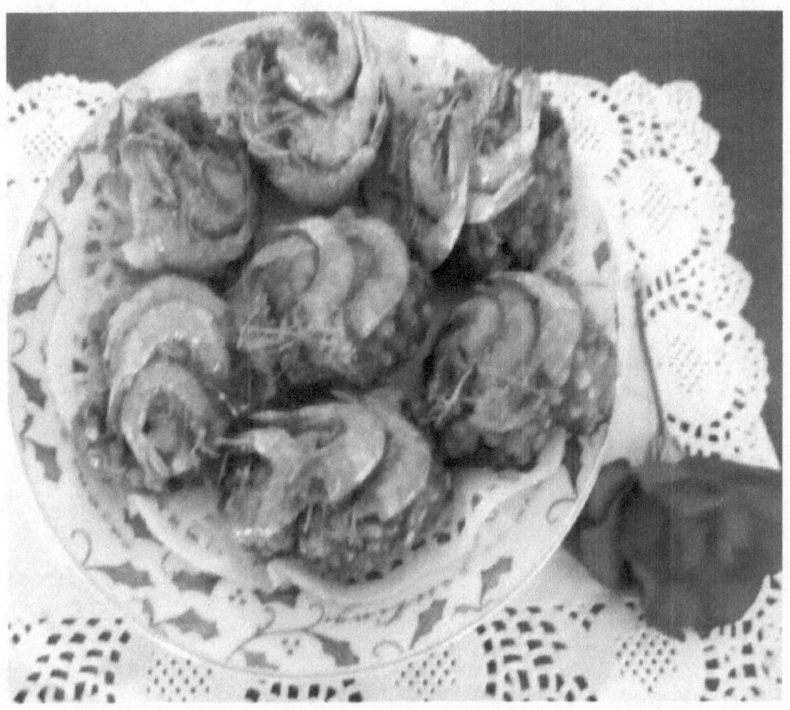

Ingredients

- 500g Red dhal (Soaked for 6 Hours and leave it to drain)
- 2 Large Onions chopped
- Curry Leaves chopped
- 7-8 Dried Chillies washed and dried
- 1 Cup of flour
- Salt
- 400g Fresh prawns –Cleaned
- 1 Tsp Chilli Powder
- ½ Bottle Coconut Oil for Frying

Method

Place the soaked dhal in a tea towel and soak well. Place the soaked dhal in a food processor and grind coarsely. Take out the mixture and add the chopped onions, salt, chilli powder and the curry leaves and mix well. If the mixture is wet add a little bit of flour and make a non-stick paste leave it a side. Mix the flour with water and make a thick paste. Make small balls from the dhal and spread on a board and apply a flour paste on top of it and add 3 or 4 prawns on top of it press firmly. Deep fry this wade in Coconut oil under slow fire until the wade turn into golden brown colour.

Masala Wade

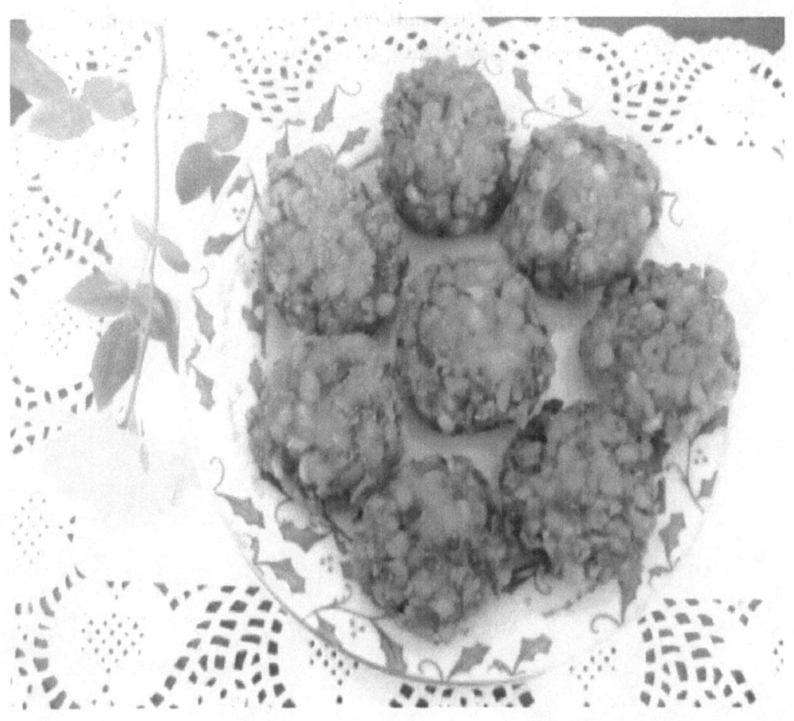

Ingredients

- 400g Chana Dhal /Chick Peas
- 1Large Onion chopped
- 8-10Curry Leaves chopped
- 2 or 3 Green Chillies chopped
- 1 tsp Chilli flakes
- ½ tsp Cumin seeds
- 2 Tsp Maldives Flakes
- Salt to taste
- ½ Bottle Coconut Oil for Frying

Method

Soak the chick peas in water for 2-3 hours, drain and grind it coarsely into a paste. Add the onions, green chilies, cumin seeds, curry leaves, chilli powder. Maldives flakes and salt .Mix well and make handful of balls .Press it using your palms and make flat chick pea patties .It shouldn't be too thin .Deep fry them in Coconut Oil until golden brown in colour in heated oil.

Ulundu Wade

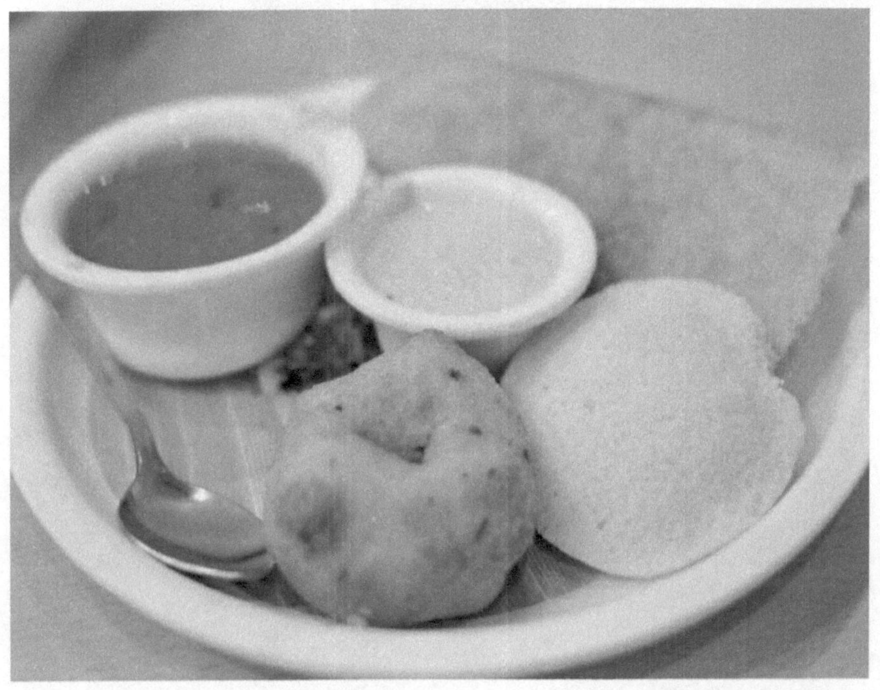

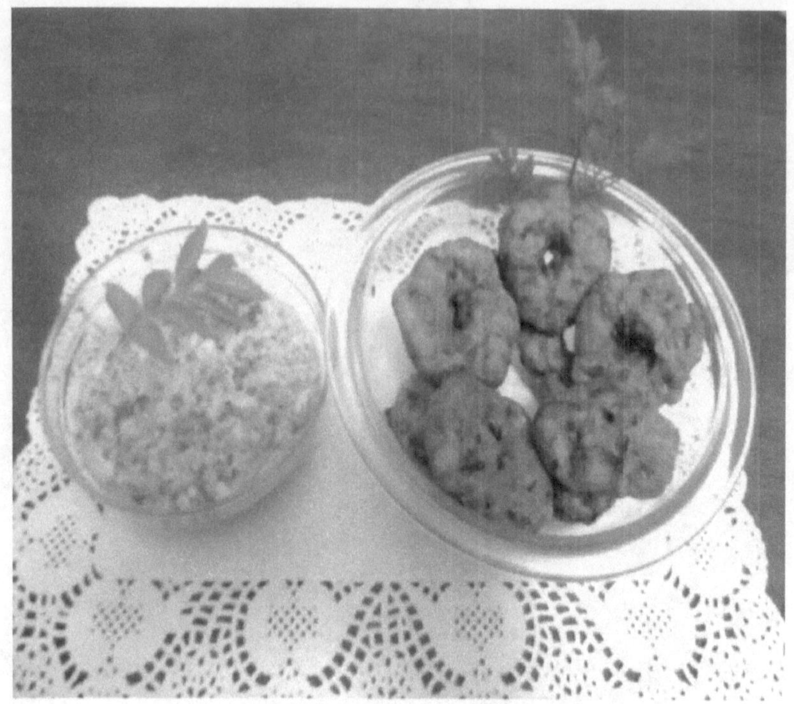

Ingredients

- 250g Ulundu Flour (Black Gram Dhal)
- 1 Onion chopped
- Green Chillies chopped
- Curry Leaves chopped
- ½ Tsp Baking Soda
- 1 Tsp Pepper
- Bit of water
- 1/2 Cup Freshly grated Coconut
- Finely lengthwise grated cabbage
- ½ Bottle Coconut oil for frying

Method

Place the Urdu flour into a mixing bowl and add curry leaves, pepper, onions, cabbage, salt to taste and ½ tsp bicarbonate and freshly grated coconut. Mix well. Add water little by little and make a thick paste. Leave for ½ hour to rise. Heat the oil. Then add some flour in your hands take a spoonful of the paste into your hand, spread it on your palm and make a whole in the middle. Deep fry in Coconut Oil until golden brown in colour. Turn both sides and fry well. Serve with Coconut Chutney.

Coconut Chutney

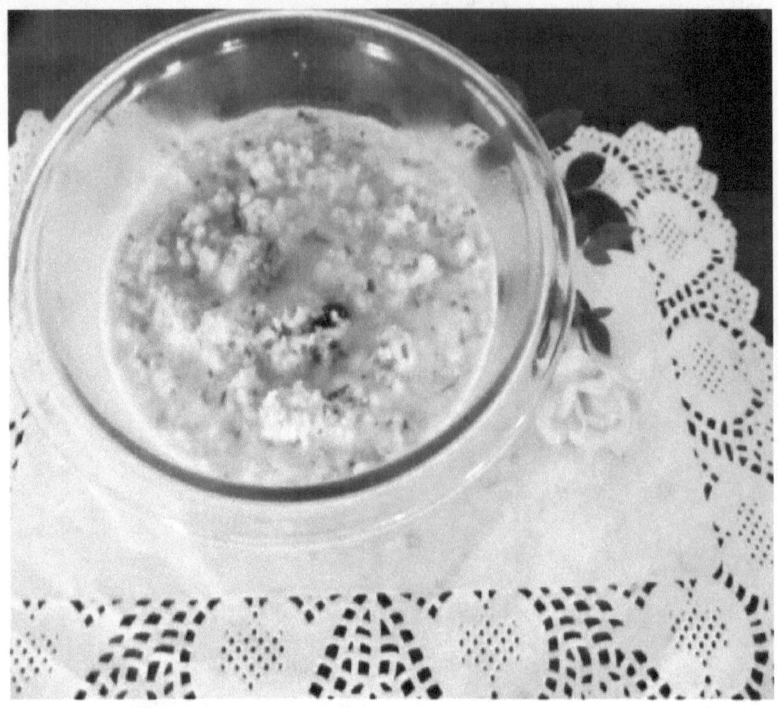

Ingredients

- 1 Cup grated Coconut
- 4-5 Green Chillies
- 1 Medium Onion
- 1 Tsp Ginger
- Salt to taste
- Pun den Leaves and Curry Leaves
- 2-3 Dried Chillies
- 2-3 Tsp Mustard Seeds
- 2 Tsp Cumin Seeds
- 2 Tbsp. Coconut Oil

Method:

Grind Onions, Green chillies well using a food processer. Then add the coconut, ginger and salt to taste and grind. Set aside the mixture. Heat 2 tbsp. Coconut oil .Add the mustard seeds, pun dun leave, curry leaves, chillies and after 2-3 minutes add the coconut mixture and temper well for 2-3 minutes and serve with wade.

Vegetable or Fish Roti (Gothamber Roti)

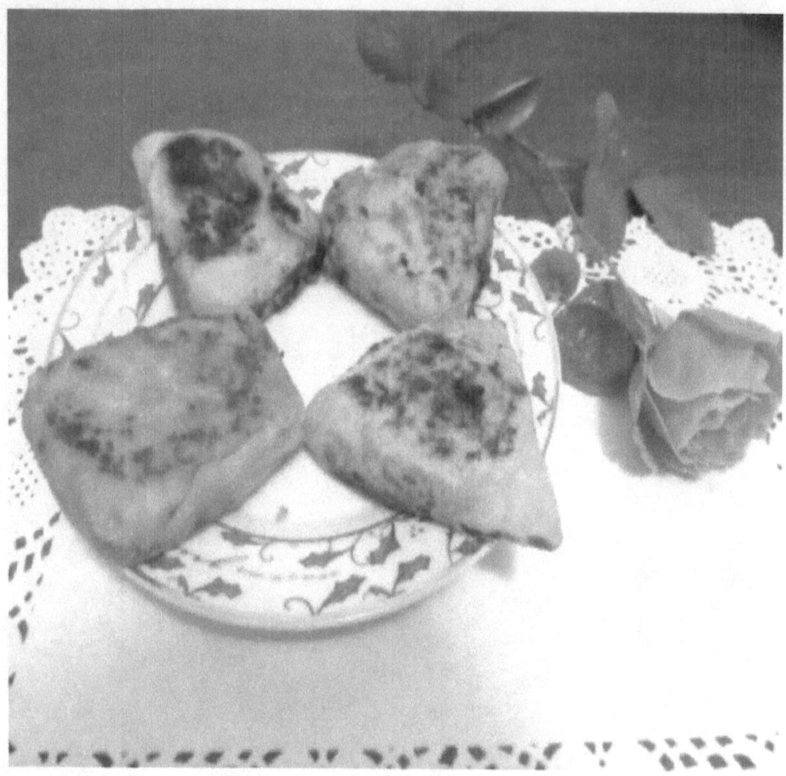

Ingredients

- 500g plain flour
- 2 tbsp. oil
- 2 cups of Luke warm water to mix
- 1 tsp Salt
- ¼ bottle Coconut Oil to dip in

Method

Place the flour in a mixing bowl and add salt. Using an electric mixer start mixing the dough. Add Luke warm water little by little and kneed it to make a smooth dough. Add about 2 tbsp. of Coconut oil to prevent the dough from sticking to the mixing bowl. Kneed the mixture for about 10 minutes until it forms a non-stick dough. After 10minutes roll the dough on a board and break into equal handful of balls. In a separate bowl place the ¼ bottle of Coconut oil and dip the ball made out of dough in the oil. Cover it using a cloth and leave it for 10 to 12 hours in the oil for good results. This will allow the oil to soak into the dough and make it smoother. But you can make it even after 1 -2 hours. Make the filling in between.

After 2 hours spread the roti and add the filling in the middle. You can shape the filling as a triangle or rectangle shape. Fold the edges into a triangle shape or rectangle shape. Heat a pan and leave it to cook on each side of the roti under a low heat. Ensure you even cook the edges. This is a yummy party food, snack as well a dinner idea.

Filling

- 1 can of Salmon or Jack mackerel-425g (or Leaks and carrots for vegetarian filling)
- 400g potatoes
- 1 big onion finely chopped
- 3 green chillies finely chopped
- 4-5 curry leaves
- 1/2 lime
- salt and pepper to taste
- ½ Tsp Chilli powder
- ½ tsp Curry Powder
- 2 Tbsp. of Coconut Oil
- Salt and Pepper

(If you don't like chilli and curry powder you can omit that and use only pepper)

Make filling: (for vegetarian recipe)

Finely chop the leeks and carrots. Mash the potatoes. Stir fry the onions in Coconut oil in a pan for about 4-5mins under low heat. Add the curry powder and chilli powder. Fry of a minute. Add the vegetables and stir fry for a few more minutes. Add the potatoes. Add salt and pepper to taste. Set aside.

Make filling: (for fish recipe)

Flake the salmon. Mash the potatoes .Stir fry the onions in Coconut oil in a pan for about 4-5mins under low heat. Add the curry powder and chilli powder. Fry of a minute. Add the fish and stir fry for a few more minutes. Add the potatoes. Add salt and pepper to taste. Set aside.

Egg Roti / Vegetarian Roti

Ingredients

- 250g plain Flour
- 1 Tsp of salt
- ½ Bottle Coconut Oil for dipping roti and 2tbs Coconut oil for frying
- 1 cups Luke warm water

Method-Dough

Add flour, Salt into an electric mixer and kneed while adding Luke warm water gradually until it forms into a non-stackable dough. After that add a little bit of Coconut oil (2 tbsp.) and mix it about 10 minutes in low speed until it form into a smooth dough.

Roll the non-sticky dough and break into small balls and dip them in a bowl of Coconut oil.

This will allow the oil to soak into the dough and make it smoother. Leave this for 12 hours covered with a damp cloth. At least 1 to 2 hours to soak the oil in to the dough.

Filling

- Leaks smoothly chopped.
- 5 Boiled potatoes
- Sliced carrot
- Chopped 1 Onions
- Chopped 2-3 Green chillies
- Pepper, Unroasted curry powder, Turmeric Powder, Chilli Powder, Roasted Curry powder, Coriander powder (If you don't like curry powder you can omit all of them)
- Salt
- Boiled Eggs
- 2 Tbsp. Coconut Oil for frying

Method

Add carrot. leaks onions, green chillies in to oil and fry. Then add the potatoes.

How to make Egg Roti

Leave a flat surface pan to heat.

After leaving the balls for 12 hours flatten the balls to a thin layer in an oiled surfaced plate. Add a big spoon full of the filling in the middle and half of an boiled egg. Shape the mixture into a rectangle and fold the edges to make a rectangle. Cook each side of the roti on the heated pan until golden brown.

Egg Sandwiches

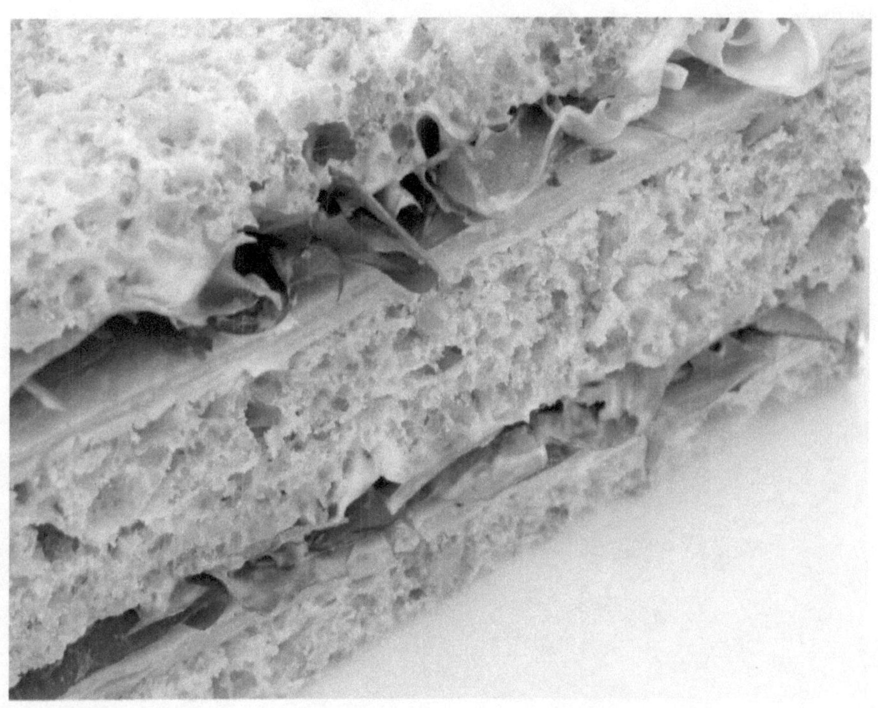

Ingredients

- 6 Hard-boiled eggs
- 1 Tsp Coconut Oil/Butter
- 3 tbsp. Mayonnaise
- Salt
- Pepper
- 1 Tsp Mustard Powder
- Parsley chopped

Method

Smash or great all the eggs. Add parsley pepper and mustard in to it. Add a little bit of salt, 3 tbsp. mayonnaise, Mix well. Spread some Butter /Coconut oil on 2 slices of bread. Spread some of the mixture on top of it and cut it into triangles.

Chicken Sandwiches

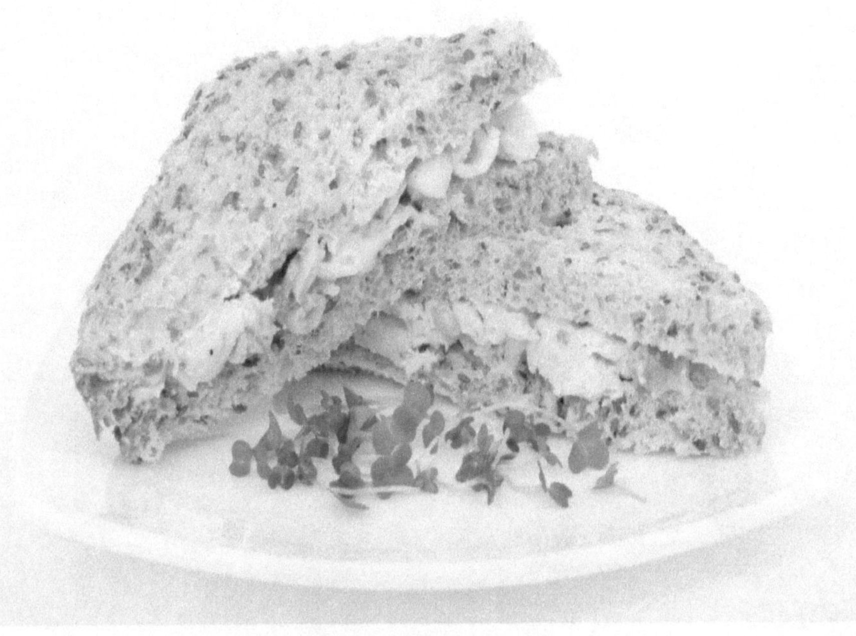

Ingredients

- 1 Chicken breast boiled in salt and peppers ½ hr
- Salt and pepper
- 1 Large onion chopped
- 2-3 Green chillies chopped
- Chopped parsley
- 2 Tbsp. Mayonnaise
- Little bit of lemon
- 1 tsp Coconut Oil

Method

Shred the boiled chicken finely into small pieces. Add bit of butter, Bit of mayonnaise, chopped parsley, Chopped onions and green chillies salt and pepper and lemon juice to taste. Apply some Coconut oil on bread and spread the filling. Cut into quarters.

Sweets

Coconut Toffee/ Coconut Rocks

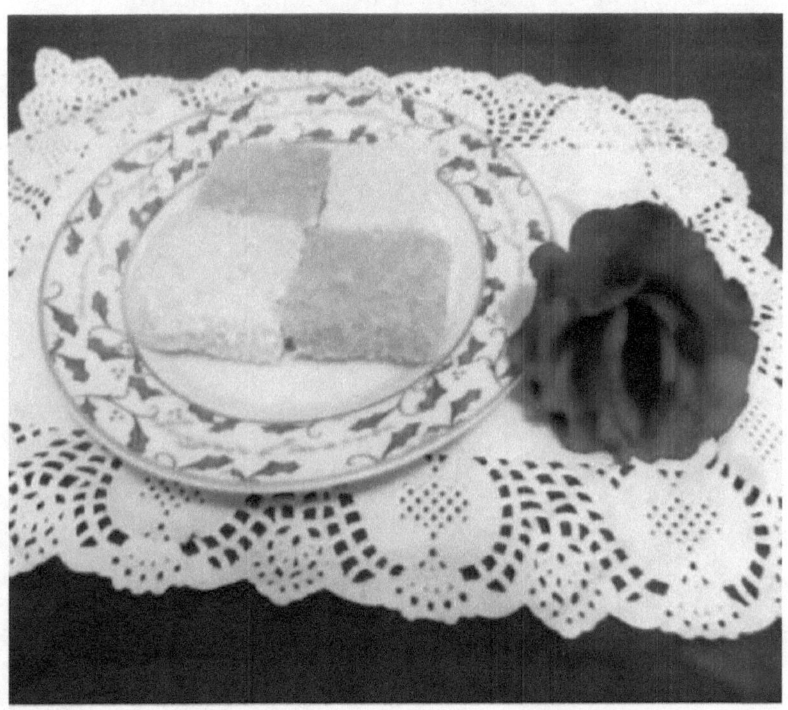

Ingredients

- 500g Desiccated coconut
- 1 Cup (220g) Sugar
- 1 Cup condensed milk
- 1 Cup Milk
- 1 Tbsp. Cardamom seeds
- 2 Tsp Vanilla Essence
- 4 Tbsp. Butter/Coconut Oil
- Pink or Green Food Colouring

Method

Butter 8 inch square Pyrex or baking tray set aside. Place non-stick pan under low heat and melt the butter in low heat .Add milk, sugar, condensed milk and let sugar dissolves .Stir .Add desiccated coconut and mix constantly for 20 minutes .Add, vanilla and pinch of food colouring and cardamoms .Mix until coconut combined together. If you like 2 separate food colourings you can separate the coconut mixture into 2 containers and add 2 separate food colourings. Transfer the mixture to the prepared Pyrex bowl/container and press firmly and set it to cool. Once it is harden a little then cut into squares using a greased knife. After cutting leave it in the refrigerator overnight to set and store in a jars .These coconut toffees will last for a week or more.

Milk Toffees / Caramel Fudge

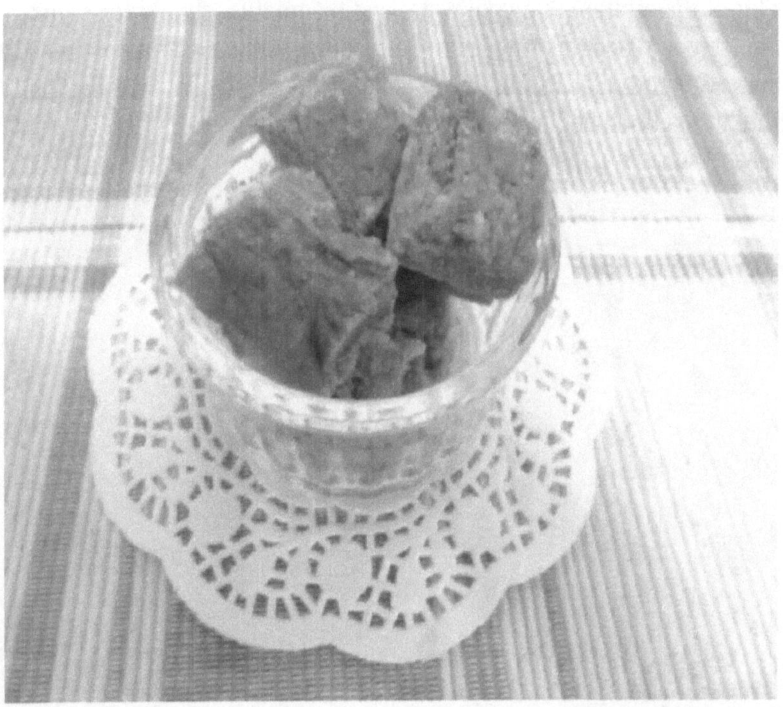

Ingredients

- 150g Coconut Oil/Butter
- 500g Brown Sugar
- 1/2 cup water
- 395 g can sweeten Condensed Milk
- 1 tsp cardamom seeds crushed
- 100g crushed cashew Nuts
- 1 Tsp Vanilla

Method

In medium heat and a heavy bottom pan stir the Condensed Milk, sugar, Coconut Oil and water. Keep on stirring until the sugar dissolves.

Continuously stir and cook for 20 minutes until the mixture thickens into a syrup that is sticky. Mixture should reach softball stage. (115 Sugar /Candy Thermometer level). If you don't have a sugar thermometer you can add a little bit of the mixture into cool water and the mixture should form into a ball. Once you reach this stage add the cashew, Vanilla, cardamom powder and mix well and remove from heat and allow the fudge to cool .Put the mixture into a lined baking tray and allow it to cool for 2-3 hours. Cut into pieces and store in jar.

Potato Toffees/ Potato Fudge

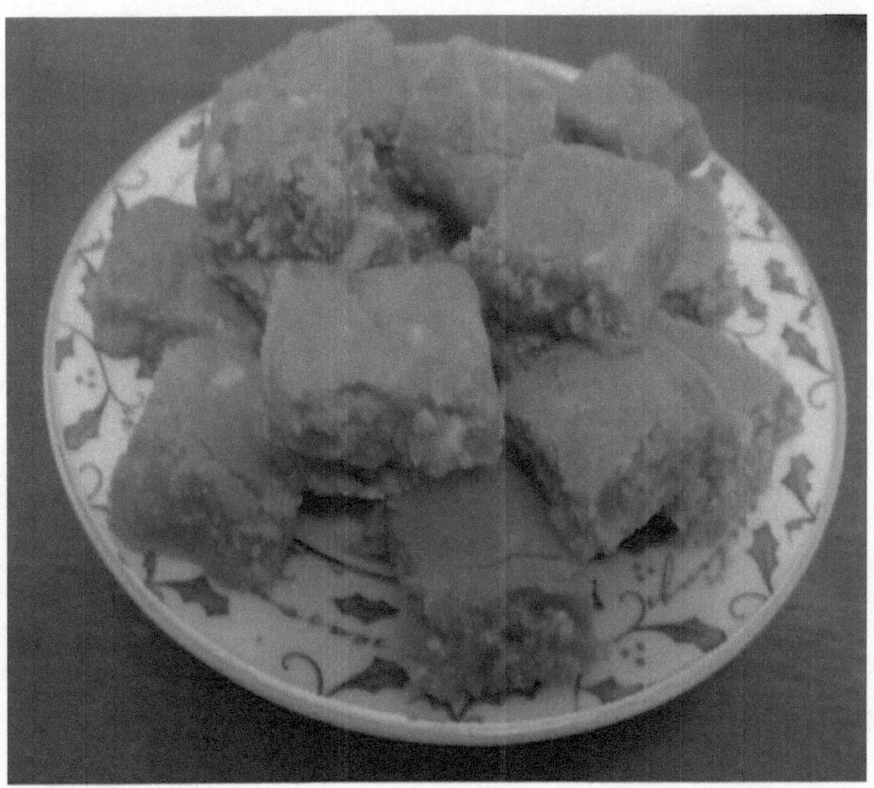

Ingredients

- 1 Tin 395G Sweeten Condensed Milk tin
- 340 g Sugar
- 125 g Butter/ Coconut Oil
- 230 g Mashed Potato's
- 100g Finely chopped Cashew Nuts
- 2 Tsp Rose Essence
- 375 ml Milk
- 1 Tsp ground Cardamoms

Directions

Put sugar, milk, condensed milk and butter or coconut oil into a large heavy bottom saucepan /Non-stick pan. Mix all together and cook over medium heat, stirring continuously. Mixture should reach softball stage or 116 degrees C (240 degrees F) on a candy thermometer. (Without a Candy thermometer softball stage can be tested by dropping a bit of the mixture into a cup of ice-cold water. If it is in the correct temperature and consistency it can be moulded into a soft ball)

Once in the softball stage remove from heat, add smoothly mashed potato and mix with a wire whisk until all lumps are beaten out. Return to heat and cook again to softball stage or 116 degrees C (240 degrees F). Then remove from heat, stir in nuts, flavouring and cardamom and mix well. Pour the mixture into a lined baked dish or into a well-buttered Pyrex dish. Press lightly with a piece of buttered banana leaf or baking paper to smooth. Cut into square pieces after 2-3 hours.

Marshmallows

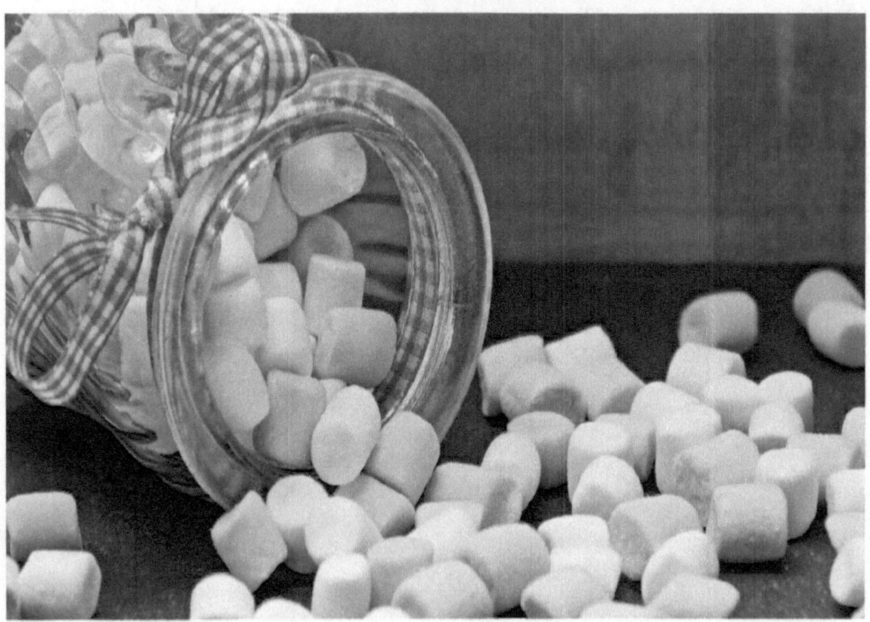

Ingredients

- 3 Tbsp. Gelatine
- ½ Cup of warm water
- 2 Cups caster sugar
- 1 Cup boiling water
- Drop of Rose water Essence
- 2-3 drops of Pink colouring
- 1 Tsp Coconut oil for spraying/lining the dish

Method

Add gelatine in the warm water and mix well and set aside to soak for 5 minutes. Put the boiled water into a pan and add the 2cups caster sugar to it.

Let the sugar dissolved completely and reach the boiling point. Boil it for 10 minutes in high heat .If low heat boil for 20 minutes. (temperature in a candy thermometer Until 140c or 200F.) Once it is dissolved take out from fire and let it cool. Spray a rectangle Pyrex bawl with coconut oil and sprinkle some icing sugar on top of it and set aside. Add the cooled gelatine syrup into an electric mixer and add the soaked gelatine into it. Beat this for about 10 minutes until the mixture turn into a fluffy consistency. Put this mixture on to the lined Pyrex bowl. If you want different colours separate into different batches and add colouring and flavour as you wish. Spread it evenly in the tray. Leave it to set outside for 3-4 hours. Do not put it in the fridge. If you like spread some icing sugar on top and let it to set. After 4 hours turn the marsh mellow upside down on to a board. Sprinkle some icing sugar on top of the base of the marsh mellow and cut into squares.

Meringues/Kisses

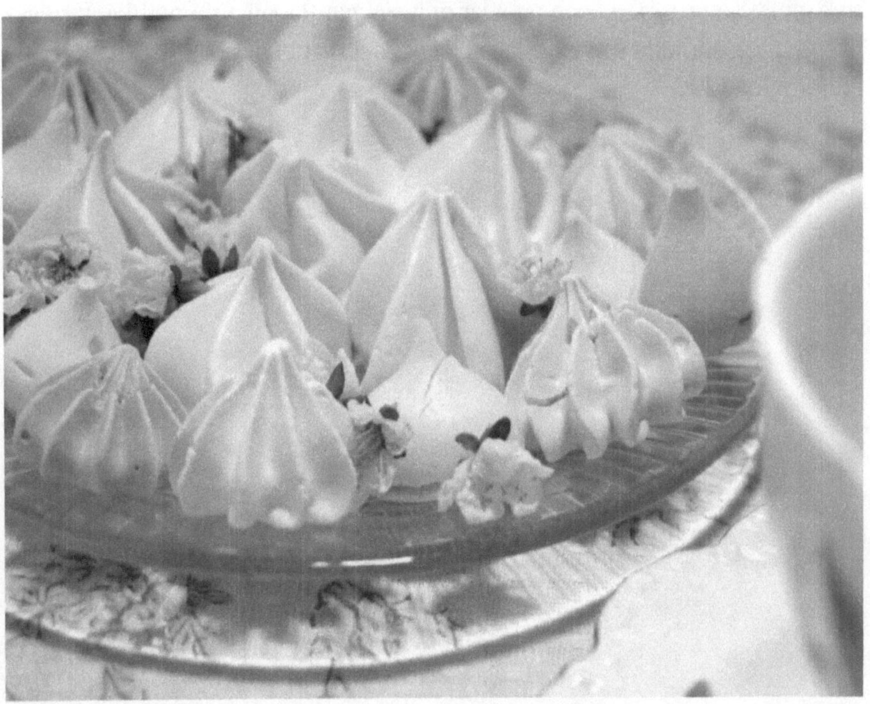

Ingredients

- 2 egg whites
- ½ cup caster sugar
- 1Tsp Vanilla/Rose Essence
- Pink/Green/Yellow drops of colouring
- 2 Tbsp. Desiccated Coconut

Method

Set the oven to 120 c .Add the egg whites in to a mixing bowl. Beat it until it forms soft peaks. Add the sugar gradually. Add vanilla into the egg white mixture and mix it for 5 minutes. Separate the egg whites into 3 separate portions and add the different colours and essence to your liking. Put the mixture into a piping bag and pipe swirls on to a baking paper. Place mixture into a piping bag fitted with a 5mm fluted or plain nozzle. Pipe 2cm wide swirls of mixture onto prepared trays, allowing 2cm between each for spreading You can add coco powder or hazel nut flavours if you like. If you like you can sprinkle some desiccated coconut on top of it and Bake it for 50 minutes for 120c.

MURRUKKU

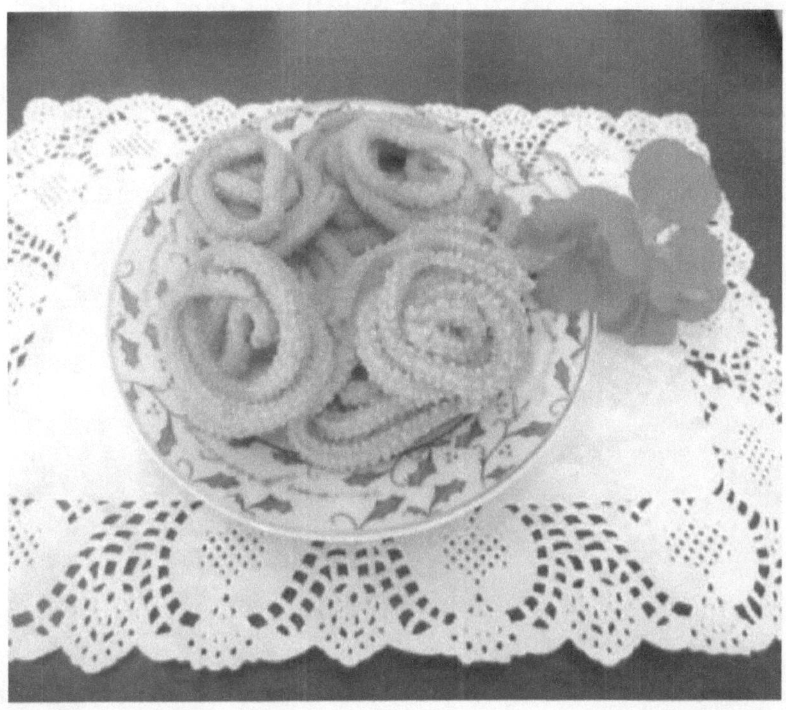

Murukku could be used as a snack or dessert. Murukku moulds with different shapes and sizes are available in most of the Indian and Sri Lankan shops.)

Ingredients:

- 1 cup kadala/chick pea flour
- 2 cups Rice flour
- 1 tsp chilli powder (optional)
- 1 tsp salt
- 2-3 cloves of garlic either crushed or ground (optional)
- 1 tsp cumin seeds (optional)
- 1 tsp of sesame seeds
- 1 Tbsp. Coconut Oil
- ½ Bottle Coconut oil for frying

Method:

Place all the above ingredients in a bowl and mix well. Add ¼-1/2 cup cold water and mix well into a thick smooth paste. Take a string hopper mould and replace with the star shape nozzle Put in the murrukku paste and make one inch size swirls in an oiled saucer and place them into the heated Coconut oil and deep fry.

You can make sugar murrukku by dipping the fried murrukku in a sugar syrup. You can make a sugar syrup with 1/2 cup of sugar, 1/8 cup of water and a few drops of vanilla. Bring it to boil. Once it is thick, take off the fire and add the prepared murukku into it and coated with sugar well.

Doughnuts

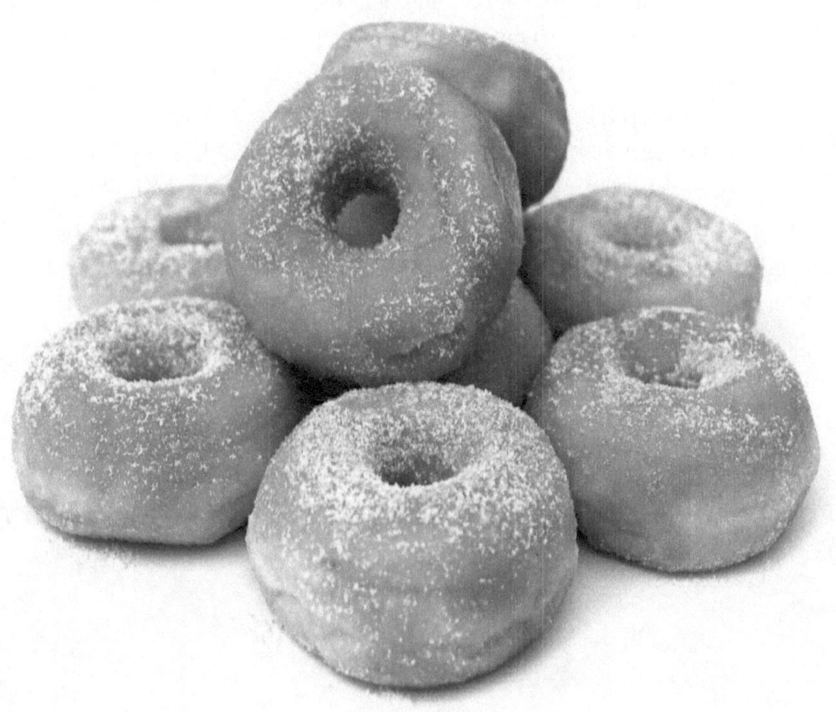

Ingredients

- 400g plain flour,
- 7g East (1 satchels)
- 1 Tsp Sugar
- 50 g castor sugar. (to sprinkle Separate)
- 1/2 tsp salt
- 30 g milk powder
- 1/2 Cup Luke warm water
- 1 Tbsp. Coconut Oil
- 100g Sugar
- 1 Egg

Mix the yeast with Luke warm water and 1 tsp of sugar. Set aside to rise. Add the plain flour ,salt , butter and milk powder in an electric mixer and knead for about 1 minute. Then add the yeast , sugar , egg. Add Luke warm water gradually and make a non-stick ball and beat for about 10-15 minutes. This will form a pliable dough.. Transfer this dough to a greased bowl and leave it to rise double in size for 40 minutes to 1 hour . After double in size transfer the dough to a floured board and roll it down to 1 cm thickness . Use a doughnut cutter and make doughnuts and place them in a baking tray and leave it further 30-40 mints to rise. Heat the oven for 160 c and bake it for 10 minutes. Take the half-baked doughnuts out and spread butter on top of them and sprinkle caster sugar on top of them. Place them again in the oven and bake again for another 7-8 minutes . You can also deep fry them in hot Coconut oil without baking. If so . Spread some melted Coconut Oil and sprinkle some caster sugar after frying.